Homemade Organic Lotion:

39 Best Natural Lotions Recipes for All Skin Types

Table of content:

Introduction

How much sense does it make to water a plastic tree? In my mind, not much. Most of what I've come across in the world of body lotions have been synthetic scientifically engineered chemicals.

Some people find such things to be fantastically useful advances in science. While I feel respect for what people today are able to do and create I remain in favor of a more natural approach to life.

It is a difficult market for those who share my sense of connection to an innate naturalistic method of living. Much of what is sold to us is composed of again, synthetic, man-engineered items. This is significant in the sense that often times such things are composed of individually toxic parts, yet as a whole avoid a dangerous level of toxicity.

The same can be said of products in the cosmetic industry. Frequently products contain elements which are not only insufficient at solving the problem they claim to, but are dangerous and harmful to the skin. Most of the time there are only trace amounts of these hazardous chemical compounds so the damage frequently occurs in the long run following extended use.

For the aforementioned reasons I strictly prefer natural lotions as they are composed of nonhazardous, naturally occurring substances. That is not to say that there are not harmful or poisonous substances that occur naturally in our environment. Yet when it comes to taking care of our skin it seems sensible to me to take advantage of the gentle solutions offered by the earth.

Natural body lotions have a greater success rate when it comes to fulfilling their promise. In most cases the particular skin type is not important as all skin benefits from some key vitamins and topical mixtures. There are also less cases of people having adverse reactions to natural body lotions. They do not contain alcohol, which severely dries the skin, and they maintain a soothing moisturizing factor that nourishes the skin.

Everyone is entitled to their own opinion but for those who are looking to take the best care of themselves they can, I say do it the natural way.

Chapter 1 – Before You Begin

Understanding Skin Types

Everybody is physically unique. In your shape, size, and composition. Everything about you is unique exactly to you—including your skin. One thing about buying lotions at the store that can be difficult is trying to find one bottle of lotion that is made for your exact skin type and meets all of your skin care needs.

Not all lotions are created equally, and with the mass marketing of brands, many skin types can get over-looked. Or, if you don't have normal skin, you may end up paying an arm and a leg for specialty lotions designed for oily or dry skin and price marked way more than they are worth.

Some lotions or creams can run upward of forty dollars. What are you paying for? More often than not, you're paying for the brand name or some expensive lab-created ingredient that does exactly the same thing as its organic counterparts.

By making your own lotion at home, you can guarantee that you create a product for the skin you have, and the skin you want. This will allow you to reap the benefits of having healthy, moisturized, hydrated skin and give you the opportunity to add some protective ingredients to prevent against environmental irritation.

While every person is unique, there are several basic categories of skin types that people fall into. Typically, after puberty you should have a pretty good idea of where you fall on the scale. If you aren't sure or if you just want to double check, read through the descriptions below and find the one that fits best with how you would describe your skin.

There are four major types of skin:

- Dry
- Normal
- Combination
- Oily

Each skin type has their own traits and attributes that can help you identify which type you have. You may not have all the traits of a certain skin type, or you may find that you have some from multiple skin type descriptions. Some skin can fall into more than one type.

Read through the descriptions and if you match more than one skin type, rank them based on how many traits you have in each category. Chances are if you only have one or two traits from a single category, then it is not enough to classify you as that primary skin type.

When making your lotion, go off your primary skin type for the area of your body that you want to use the lotion on. If your face identifies as one skin type but your body is another, then you may need to make two lotions: one for your face and one for your body. That way your skin gets the best treatment based on the primary type it aligns with.

Dry skin if you suffer from dry skin you can identify this condition by the following traits:

- Small pores which are almost unnoticeable
- Red, patchy skin
- Itchy skin
- Cracked skin
- Peeling skin

Dry skin can be a result of genetics, medication, or a medical condition. Treating dry skin is important to maintain skin elasticity, comfort, and prevent other possible heath conditions.

Normal Skin Normal skin can be identified by the following traits:

- Few imperfections or blemishes
- Small pores which are barely visible
- Minimal sensitivity or no severe sensitivity

Most people will have normal skin after puberty. This has a light, healthy layer of oils that keep the skin lightly moisturized and gives a "radiant" appearance.

Combination Skin Combination skin affects the highest percentage of individuals. Combination skin means having more than one skin type.

Typically, this can be identified if you have patches of dry or oily skin and patches of normal skin. This can look like normal skin with an oily T-zone on your face, or normal skin all over with patches of dry skin on your arms, *etc.*

Traits of Combination Skin are:

- Noticeable or dilated pores
- Blackheads
- "Shiny" or an oily sheen on the skin
- Spots of red, patchy skin

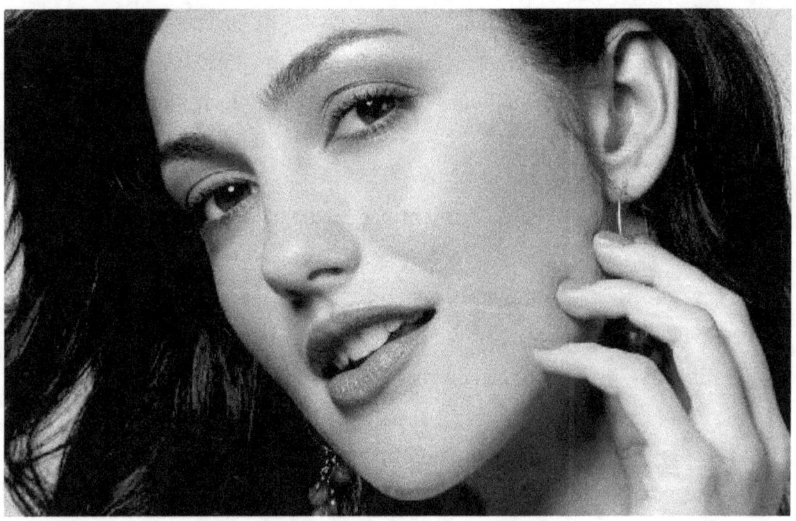

Combination skin can be treated by making two different types of lotion, or by focusing on whichever skin type is more dominant. If your skin is oilier than it is normal or dry, then focus on that skin type.

Oily Skin Oily skin is very common for individuals going through puberty and some adults. This is because the change in hormones can result in the body producing more oil for the skin.

Traits of oily skin are:

- Oversized or enlarged pores
- A thick oily sheen or "shine" to the skin
- Acne, blackheads, and clogged pores
- A feeling of "heaviness" to the skin due to the exaggerated oil production.

If you have oily skin it is important to clean your skin regularly to prevent dirt and grime from getting trapped in the pores. Hydrating the skin can help keep it healthy. Avoid drying out the skin unless you are treating on-the-spot acne. Drying out oily skin too much can result in other skin conditions.
Once you have identified the type of skin you have, it will make the process of selecting what type of lotion to make that much easier. You may find that it is best for you to make multiple lotion types for different areas of the skin.

Base Ingredients of the Lotion.

Lightweight lotion oils: This is best if you are making a lotion for any skin type.

- Olive Oil

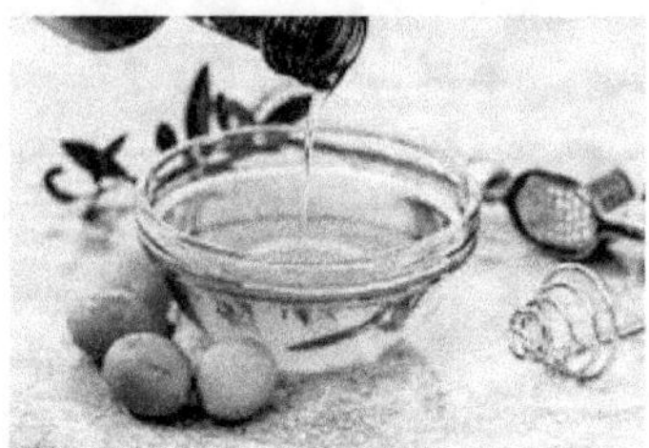

Olive oil has antioxidants and Vitamin E in it to protect your skin from premature aging, ultraviolet rays, and skin damage. It also doesn't clog pores and it enhances exfoliation to clear away dead skin cells. This is great for all skin types.

- Almond Oil

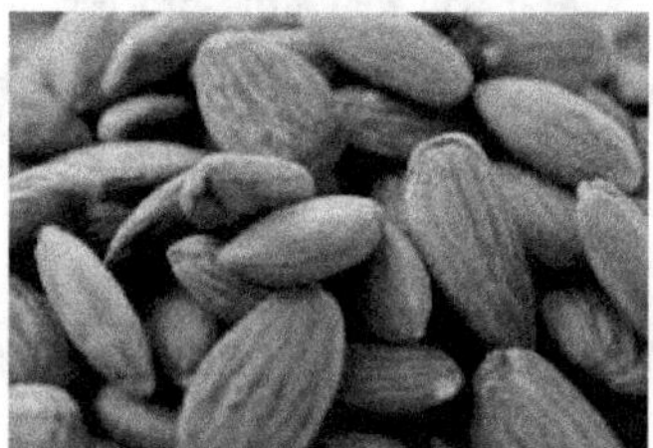

Almond oil is hypoallergenic (provided you do not have a nut allergy ;) it has Vitamin A to help clean the pores, remove dirt, and reduce acne; it can relieve irritation to the skin due to sun exposure; and it can help treat eczema. This is great for normal to dry skin.

- Coconut Oil

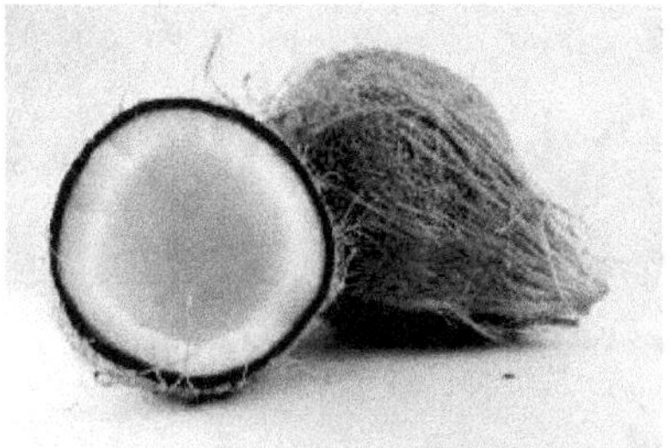

Coconut oil has saturated fats which help retain moisture in the skin. It also has Vitamin E which protects the skin from ultraviolet rays, premature aging, and skin damage. This is great for all skin types.

- Avocado Oil

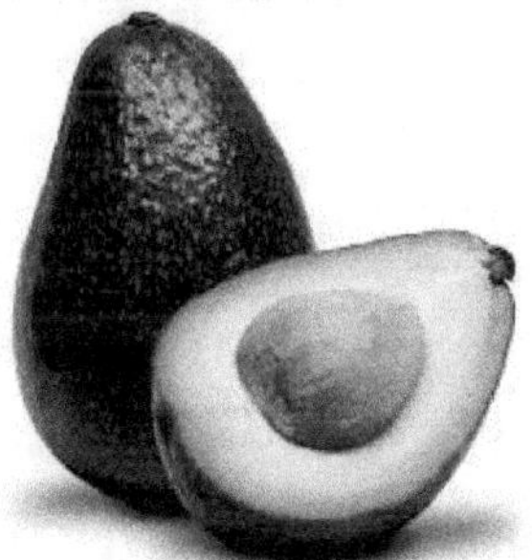

Avocado oil is high in nutrients and vitamin which are valuable to the skin. It enhances the natural ability for the skin to create collagen, which is what retains the skin's elasticity and firmness. The proteins and fats in the oil help keep the skin moisturized which can help treat eczema and other dry skin issues. This is great for normal to dry skin.

- Apricot Oil

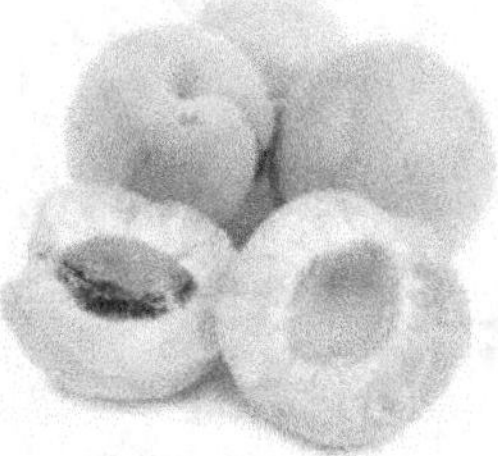

Apricot oil is great for normal skin, oily skin, and hormonal skin. It is gentle and does not leave an oily residue or coat on the skin. Because of this, it is great for the face or oily skin due to its lightness.

Heavy weight butters these are best for body butters or creams for normal to dry skin, or if you want long lasting moisture without needing to reapply.

- Cocoa Butter

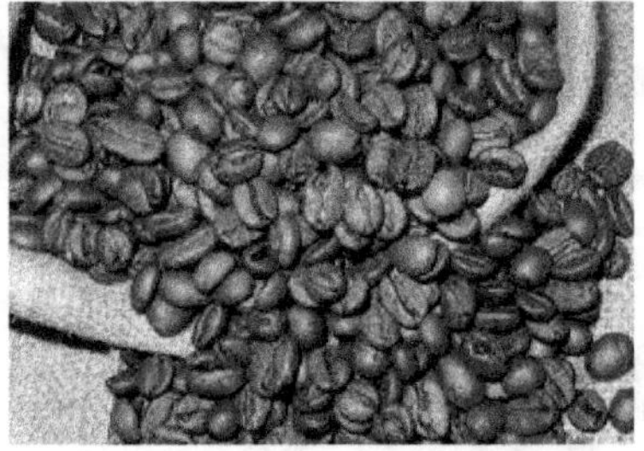

Cocoa butter is a good replacement to use if you have any nut allergies. Cocoa butter is thick, and gentle on the skin. It is pure vegetable fat harvested from the cocoa bean. The fat in cocoa butter helps the skin retain moisture and it works to smooth the skin and has anti-aging properties, as well. It is also rich in antioxidants which protect the skin from damage caused by ultraviolet rays and other external factors that can cause skin irritation or harm.

- Shea Butter

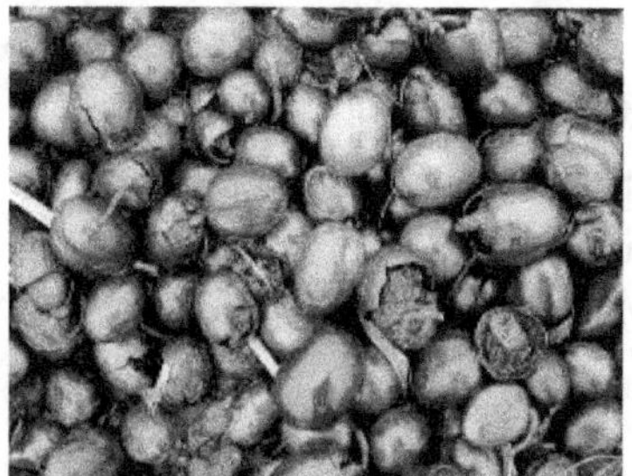

Shea butter is the most common ingredient in heavy weight body butters. Shea butter not only moisturizes skin, but the nutrients and vitamins in it help to restore collagen for skin elasticity. Shea butter also works as an anti-inflammatory for irritated skin, it reduces stretch marks, protects skin from ultraviolet rays, and is gentle enough on the skin that it can be used on babies. If you have nut allergies, don't use Shea butter, but opt for cocoa butter instead.

If you want to make a mid-weight cream, combine one of the lightweight oils with a small amount of one of the butters. This will thicken the lotion just enough to make it a cream, without adding all the weight of a body butter.

There are several different types of lotion and each one has its own function and purpose. Based on your skin type, and the needs of your skin that you're hoping your homemade organic lotion will help with, you may need to make a certain kind of lotion or several to meet a variety of needs.

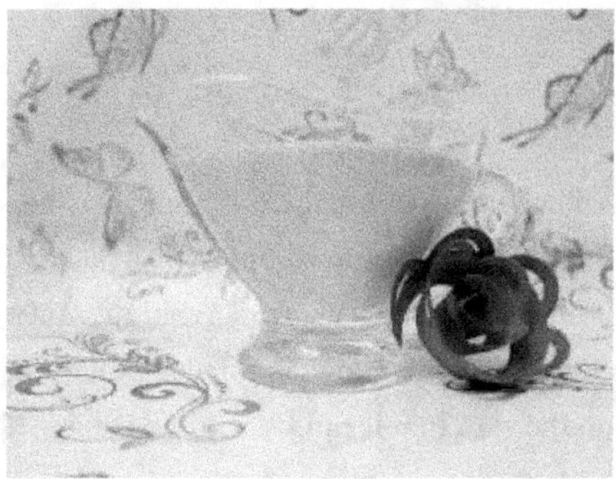

There are two main types of lotion that you can easily make at home:

- Generic lotion
- Body butter

Each type of lotion has a different function and a different base to give it a specific weight. When discussing "weight" as it pertains to a lotion, the weight corresponds with how thick the lotion is. The lighter it is, the faster it absorbs and the more likely you are going to need to reapply it. The thicker it is, the longer it will sit on the skin to moisturize it.

There are pros and cons to each weight, and those will depend on your skin type and your everyday needs.

Lightweight A lightweight lotion is going to have a light oil base and will blend easily into the skin. It will typically absorb right away, or within a few minutes. This can be nice if you can't afford oily or greasy hands or appendages, but it also means you will need to reapply more frequently.

A lightweight lotion is great for people with oily skin who do not need a lot of extra moisturizer, but still want to give their skin the extra nutrients and benefits that come with moisturizing.

Lightweight lotions are also great for hands. Lightweight lotion is good to use for your hands because if you use your hands a lot at work, and depending on what you do, you might not be able to afford oily or greasy hands which can happen if you use a lotion that is too heavy.

Lightweight lotions are also perfect to use on your face because you don't want anything too heavy that could clog your pores and lead to acne. A nice, lightweight lotion will moisturize your skin and help with the appearance of wrinkles as well as preventing breakouts. Although it is a common misconception that oil=acne, moisturized and hydrated skin can actually prevent breakouts. This is because well-moisturized skin has a healthy layer of oil which protects against dryness and dirt which can lead to clogged pores and result in acne. Too much oil can also trap dirt, which is why cleaning and washing your face regularly is important.

Mid-weight A mid-weight lotion is good for normal or combination skin. Combination skin is where you have both oily and normal or dry skin. This can result in specific spots where your skin is oilier—like an oily T-zone.

Mid-weight lotions will absorb into the skin a little more slowly than a lightweight lotion, but won't stay on the skin as long as a heavier butter. This is why having a mid-weight lotion or cream is great for the hands or body.

Heavy weight A heavy weight lotion is also known as a butter or cream. This might be more recognizable as a body butter. Heavy lotions or butter stay on the skin for long periods of time. While this can be troublesome if you have it on your hands because it will leave an oily or greasy residue for a while until it is absorbed completely into the skin, it also works the best because it lasts the longest and provides your skin with long-lasting moisture and hydration.

Body butters or heavy lotions are great for using on the body and extremities such as the arms or legs. It will go on thick and slowly absorb into the skin throughout the day or night (depending on when you put it on.) Heavy lotions or body butters are great for people with dry skin or chronic dry skin because it will provide a layer of moisture on top of the skin while it soaks in. It is also good to use for people with normal or combination skin.

Heavy lotions or butters can be too much for people with oily skin. Adding this additional moisture to already oily skin can result in a greasy feeling, a heaviness to the skin, and clogged pore which can lead to acne.

If you're not sure what skin type you have, you can test each lotion weight on a patch of skin to find out. It is recommended to test on a patch of skin on your arm where it can be easily washed if you do not like the result of the product.

The great thing about making your own lotion is that you can make it to fit your exact skin type.

More details will be provided in Chapters 3 and 4, but it is best to start with the lightweight lotion and then add more ingredients as needed to make it mid-weight (cream) or heavy weight (butter).

Chapter 2 – Lotions for Dry Skin

Pumpkin Spice Lotion

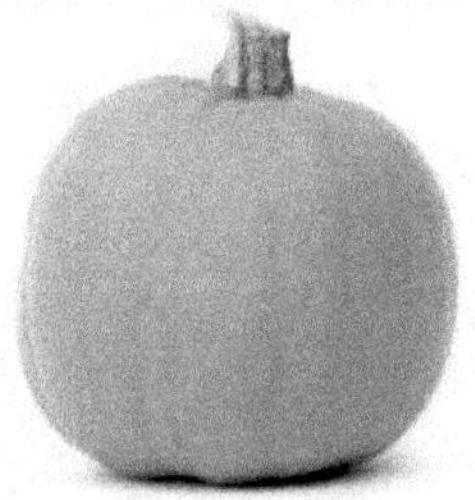

Ingredients:

- 8 ounces of shea butter
- 2 cups of coconut oil
- 20 drops of pumpkin spice essential oil

Directions:

1. Melt the coconut oil with shea butter in a double boiler then remove it from the heat while some soft chunks of butter are still visible.

2. Blend the mix with a stand mixer until it becomes smooth and creamy then add in the essential oil and blend it again.

3. Transfer the lotion into mason jars and secure their lids then allow it to cool down completely.

4. Apply this lotion to your body whenever you desire.

5. This lotion smells heavenly and softens your skin at the same time.

Creamy Coconut Aloe Vera Lotion

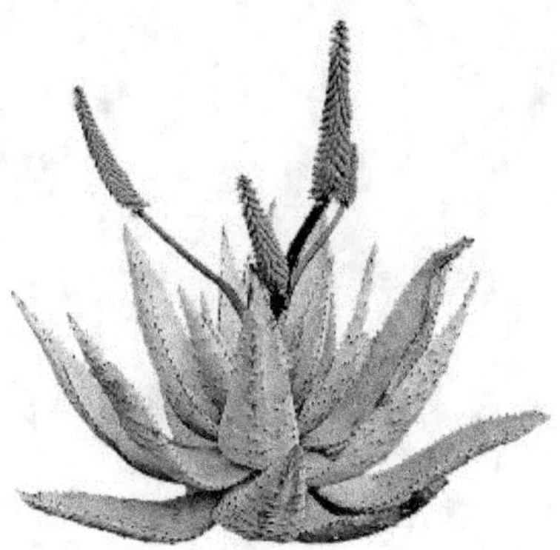

Ingredients:

- ¼ cup of solid coconut oil
- 1 teaspoon of aloe vera gel
- 3 drops of rose essential oil
- 2 drops of lavender essential oil

Directions:

1.   Beat the coconut oil using a hand mixer until it becomes creamy then stir into it the essential oil and aloe vera gel.

2.   Transfer the lotion to a mason jar and seal the lid then use it right away or refrigerate it.

3.   After an eventful day, this lotion will help you relax your sore muscles.

Creamy Jojoba Lotion

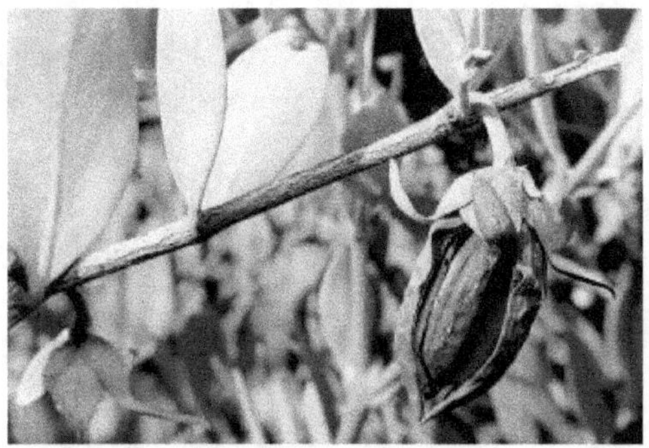

Ingredients:

- 1 cup of cold pressed coconut oil
- 1 cup of pure shea butter
- 2 tablespoons of vegetable glycerin
- 1 tablespoon of jojoba oil

Directions:

1. Combine all the ingredients in a food processor and blend them smooth then transfer the mix to a bowl and refrigerate it until it solidifies.

2. Once the time is up, whip the lotion with a hand mixer until it becomes creamy.

3. Apply this lotion to your body whenever you desire.

4. This lotion is nourishing; it will smoothen and soften your skin.

Grapefruit Body Lotion

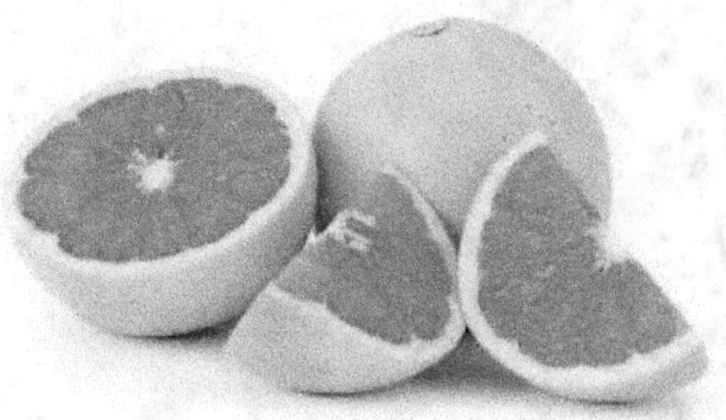

Ingredients:

- ½ cup of coconut oil
- The zest of 1 red grapefruit
- 2 tablespoons of raw shea butter
- 2 teaspoons of tapioca starch
- 2 drops of almond essential oil

Directions:

1. Combine the coconut oil with shea butter and grapefruit zest in a bowl and beat them for 30 sec on medium then turn it on high and whip it for another 4 min.

2. Once the time is up, add in the rest of the ingredients and whip them for another 30 sec.

3. Apply this lotion to your body whenever you desire.

4. This lotion will nourish and moisturize your skin.

Lavender Arrow Lotion

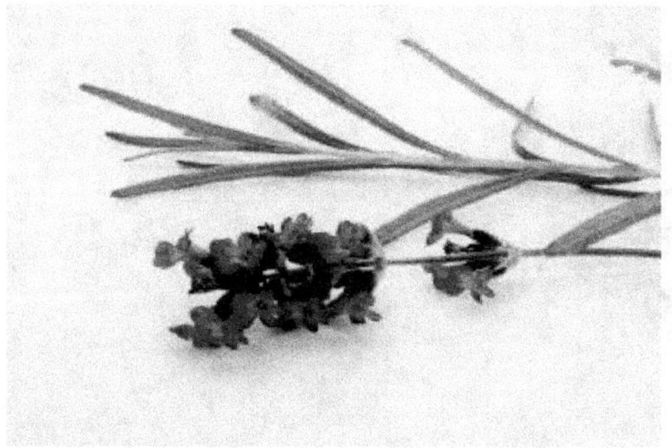

Ingredients:

- 1 cup of coconut oil
- 1 cup of raw shea butter
- 1/3 cup of arrowroot powder
- 100 drops of lavender essential oil

Directions:

1. Combine all the ingredients in a medium bowl and whip them until their soft peaks.

2. Transfer the mix into a mason jar and seal it then use it right away or refrigerate it until ready to use.

3. If you want a creamy lotion that moisturizes your skin without making it greasy, this lotion is perfect for you.

Woodsy Myrrh Lotion

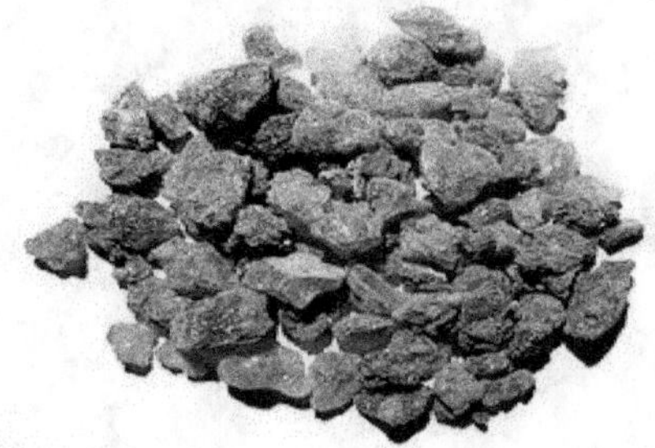

Ingredients:

- ¼ cup of coconut oil
- ¼ cup of raw shea butter
- ¼ cup of olive oil
- ¼ cup of beeswax
- 20 drops of myrrh essential oil
- 20 drops of frankincense essential oil

Directions:

1. Combine all the ingredients in a double boiler except for the essential oils and stir them until they completely melt.

2. Remove the mix from the heat and sit in the essential oils then whip them until they become fluffy and creamy.

3. Transfer the mix into a mason jar and seal it then use it right away or refrigerate it until ready to use.

4. This lotion with make your skin soft and smooth like a baby's.

Chapter 3 – Lotions for Normal Skin

Minty Aloe Vera Lotion

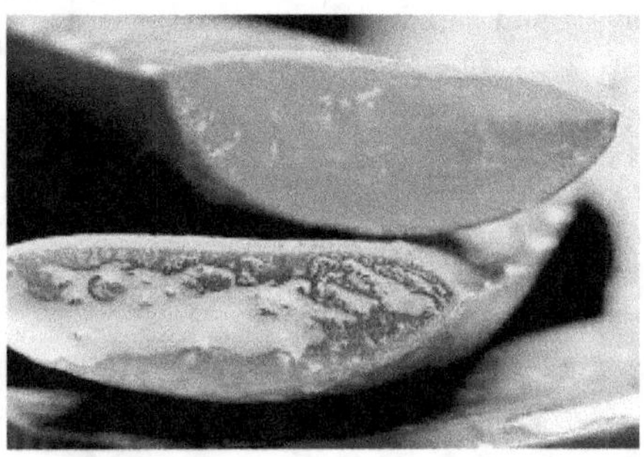

Ingredients:

- ½ cup of aloe vera gel
- ½ cup of coconut oil
- ¼ cup of beeswax, grated
- 1/8 teaspoon of peppermint oil

Directions:

1.   Melt the wax with coconut oil in a double boiler then remove it from the heat.

2.   Add in the peppermint oil with aloe vera gel and whisk them until they become smooth.

3.   Place the lotion in an ice bath and stir it until it becomes creamy and slightly thick then allow it to cool down for 1 h.

4.   Once the time is up, transfer the lotion to a food processor and blend it for 30 sec.

5.   Transfer the mix into a mason jar and seal it then use it right away or refrigerate it until ready to use.

6.   This lotion will be sooth your skin and repairs all the damage that the sun caused to it.

Floral Lotion

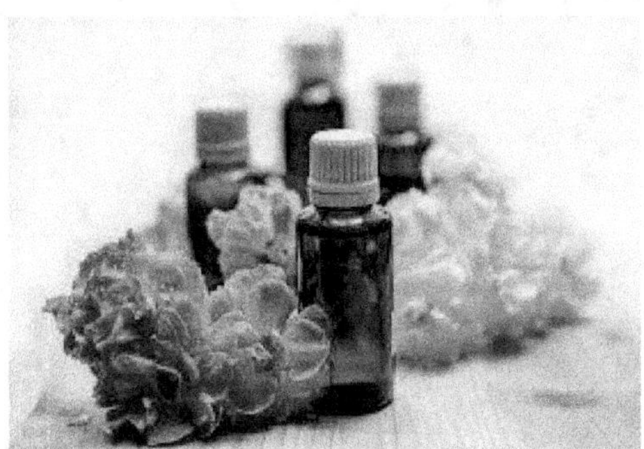

Ingredients:

- ½ cup of orange floral water
- ¾ cup of grapeseed oil
- ¼ cup of distilled water
- ½ ounce of beeswax
- 8 drops of lavender essential oil
- 8 drops of orange essential oil

Directions:

1.   Melt the wax with grapeseed oil in a double boil then remove it from the heat and allow it to cool down until it becomes warm to the touch.

2.   Stir in the distilled water with orange floral water then transfer them to a food processor and blend them smoothly.

3.   Add in the essential oils to the lotion mix and blend them for 30 sec.

4.   Transfer the lotion into a mason jar and seal it then use it right away or refrigerate it until ready to use.

5.   You can use this lotion every day especially if you have dry skin, and you can use it on your babies as well.

Nutty Roses Lotion

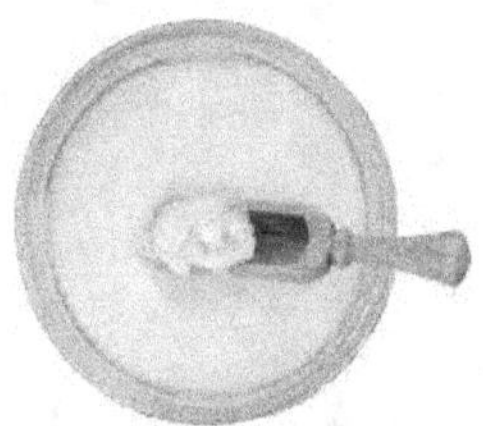

Ingredients:

- 1 cup of raw shea butter
- ½ cup of coconut oil
- ½ cup of sweet almond oil
- 5 drops of carrot seed essential oil
- 5 drops of rosemary essential oil

Directions:

1.   Melt the almond oil with butter and coconut oil in a double boiler then stir in the essential oils right away.

2.   Chill the lotion in the fridge for 2 h until it hardens then whip it with a hand mixer until it becomes creamy and soft.

3.   Transfer the lotion into a mason jar and seal it then use it right away or refrigerate it until ready to use.

4.   This lotion will keep your skin moisturized and soft the whole day.

Lavender Roses Lotion

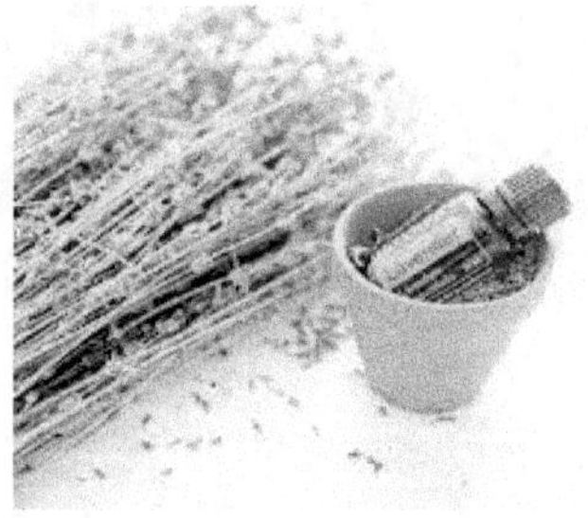

Ingredients:

- 16 ounces of baby lotion
- 8 ounces of Vitamin E cream
- 8 ounces of Vaseline
- 5 drops of rose essential oil
- 5 drops of lavender essential oil

Directions:

1.   Combine all the ingredients in a mixing bowl then whip them until they become creamy.

2.   Transfer the lotion into a mason jar and seal it then use it right away or refrigerate it until ready to use.

3.   This is an incredible moisturizing lotion that will leave your skin smelling heavenly.

Frankincense Vanilla Lotion

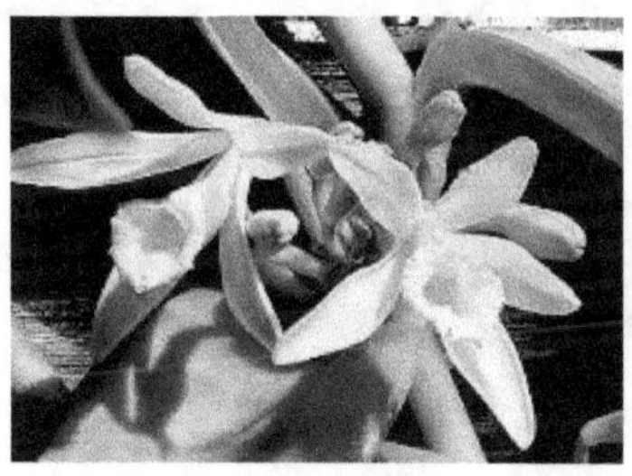

Ingredients:

*   1 cup of olive oil
*   ¼ cup of beeswax
*   ¼ cup of coconut oil
*   2 tablespoons of cocoa butter
*   1 teaspoon of vitamin E oil
*   5 drops of vanilla essential oil
*   5 drops of frankincense essential oil

Directions:

1.   Stir all the ingredients in the bowl of a double boiler.

2.   Transfer the lotion into a mason jar and seal it then use it right away or refrigerate it until ready to use.

3.   This is an incredible moisturizing lotion that will leave your smelling skin heavenly.

Lavender Lemon Lotion

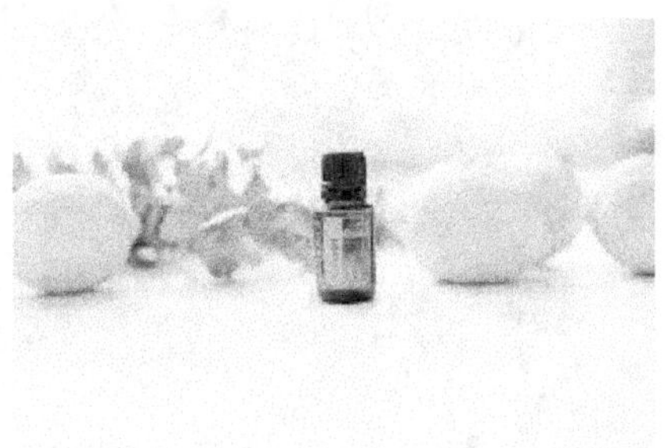

Ingredients:

- 1 cup of aloe vera gel
- ½ cup of sweet almond oil
- ½ cup of beeswax, grated
- 1 teaspoon of vitamin E oil
- 5 drops of lavender essential oil
- 5 drops of lemon essential oil
- 5 drops of Eucalyptus essential oil

Directions:

1.   Whisk the aloe vera gel with vitamin E oil and almond oil in a small bowl then set it aside.

2.   Melt the beeswax in a double boiler then pour it in a food processor and add to it the oils and aloe vera mix.

3.   Cover the processor and blend them smooth then add in the essential oils and blend them again until you get a creamy mix.

4.   This lotion will repair and moisturize your skin, especially in the harsh winter.

Tea Carrot Lotion

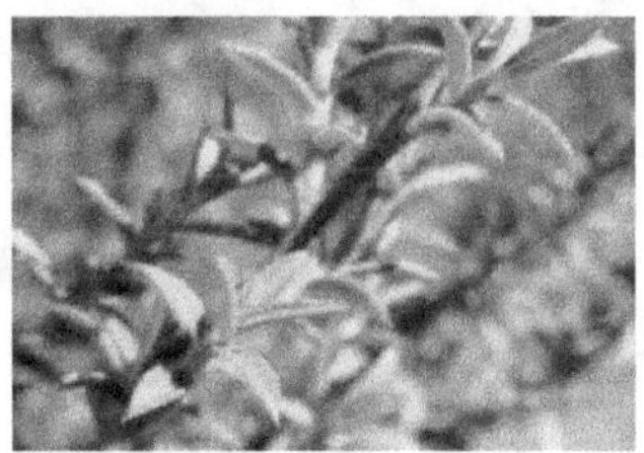

Ingredients:

- 4 ounces of shea butter
- 2 tablespoons of avocado oil
- 10 drops of lavender essential oil
- 5 drops of carrot seed oil
- 5 drops of tea tree essential oil
- 5 drops of rosemary essential oil

Directions:

1.   Place the butter in a saucepan and melt it over low heat then stir into it the avocado oil and remove it from the heat.

2.   Refrigerate the mix for 15 to 20 min until it starts to harden.

3.   Once the time is up, add in the essential oils to the mix and whip them until they become light and creamy.

4.   Transfer the lotion into a mason jar and seal it then use it right away or refrigerate it until ready to use.

5.   This is an incredible moisturizing lotion will nourish your skin and provide with all the vitamins that it needs.

Chamomile Lotion Bar

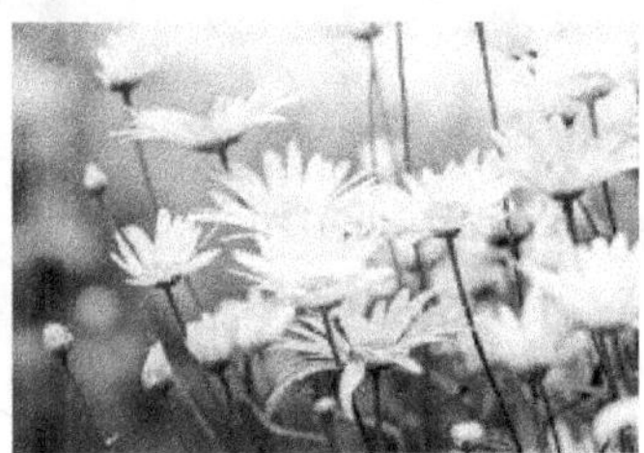

Ingredients:

- 1/8 cup of coconut oil
- 2 1/8 tablespoons of cocoa butter
- 1 1/3 tablespoon of beeswax

- 1 teaspoon of peppermint essential oil
- ½ teaspoon of lavender essential oil
- ¼ teaspoon of rosemary essential oil
- 15 drops of chamomile essential oil

Directions:

1.   Combine the beeswax with cocoa butter and coconut oil in a double boiler and stir them until they completely.

2.   Remove the oils from the heat and stir into it the essential oils.

3.   Transfer the lotion into a mason jar and seal it then use it right away or refrigerate it until ready to use.

4.   This lotion is an amazing moisturizer for your skin; you can use it for your baby as well without worrying about anything.

Chapter 4 – Lotions for Oily Skin

Tropical Creamy Lotion

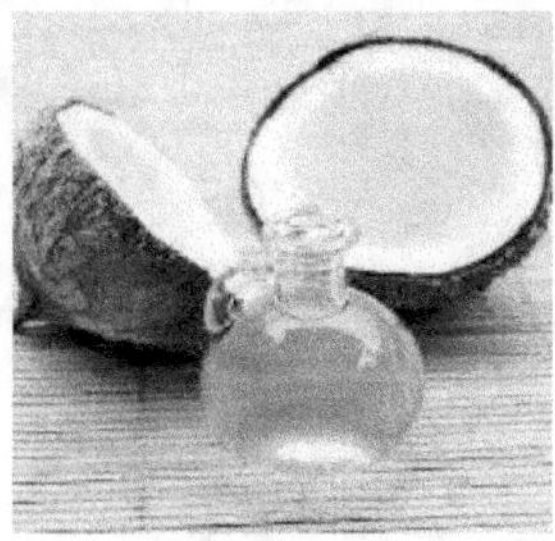

Ingredients:

- ½ cup of coconut oil
- ½ cup of shea butter
- 10 drops of orange essential oil
- 10 drops of lime essential oil
- 5 drops of grapefruit essential oil

Directions:

1.   Melt the shea butter with coconut oil in a double boiler and allow it to cool down for 3 to 5 min.

2.   Add in the essential oils and whip the mix until it becomes creamy then use it after shaving and enjoy.

3.   This lotion will make your skin so soft and fresh not to mention that it will stop the itching feeling that you get after shaving.

Bluish Winter Lotion

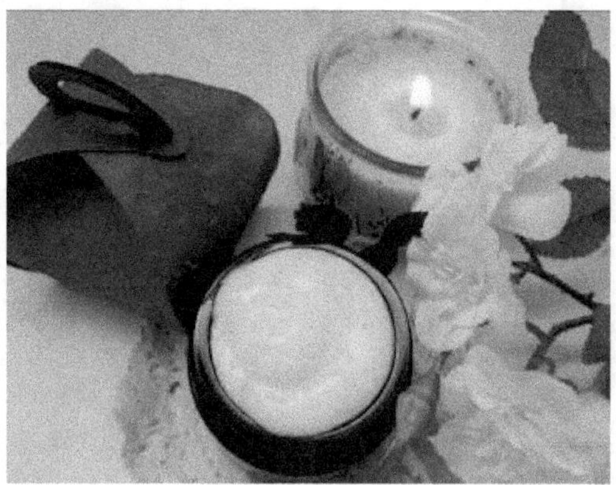

Ingredients:

- 27 ounces of baby lotion
- 8 ounces of coconut oil
- 7 ounces of Aquaphor
- 4 ounces of Fruit of Earth vitamin E cream

Directions:

1.   Combine all the ingredients in a large bowl and whip them with a hand mixer until they become creamy.

2.   Transfer the mix into a mason jar and refrigerate it then use it whenever you desire.

3.   This lotion is perfect for the harsh winter season that leaves your skin chapped and cracked, this lotion will repair your skin and keep it moisturized.

Lavender Facial Lotion

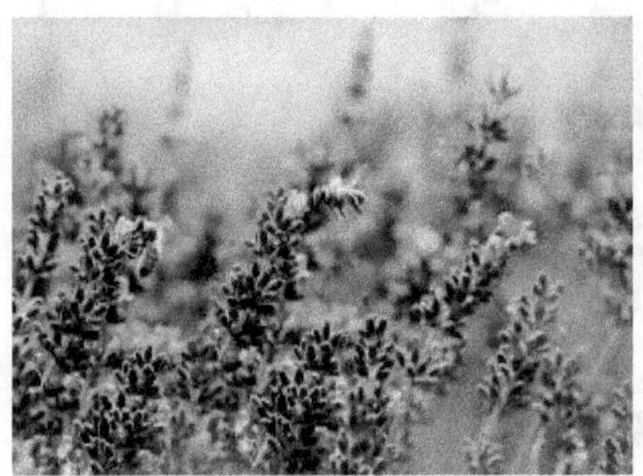

Ingredients:

- 3 ½ tablespoons of shea butter
- 3 tablespoons of ale vera gel
- 2 tablespoons of jojoba oil
- 1 teaspoon of vitamin E oil
- 4 drops of lavender essential oil

Directions:

1. Melt the jojoba oil with butter in a double boiler then stir into them the aloe vera gel and whip them until they become creamy.

2. Add in the rest of the ingredients and whip them for 1 min then transfer the lotion into a mason jar and use it whenever you desire.

3. This lotion is perfect for people that have dry skin; it will leave your skin moisturized and soft.

Creamy Magnesium Lotion

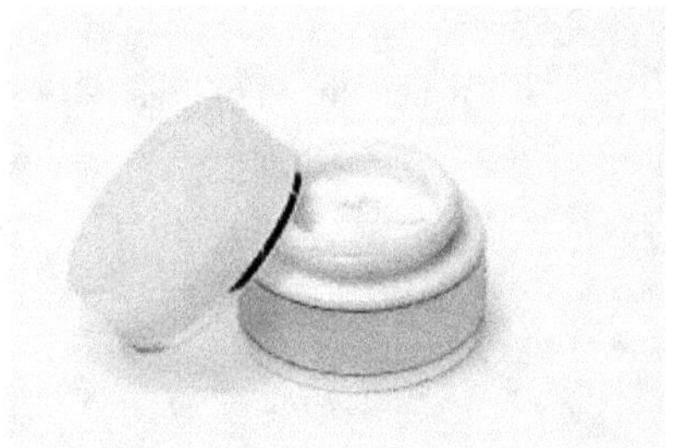

Ingredients:

- ½ cup of magnesium flakes
- ¼ cup of grapes seeds oil
- ¼ cup of coconut oil
- 3 tablespoons of distilled water
- 2 ½ tablespoons of beeswax, grated
- 1 tablespoon of shea butter
- 1 teaspoon of vitamin E oil
- 20 drops of lavender essential oil
- 10 drops of peppermint essential oil

Directions:

1.   Bring the water to a boil then remove it from the heat and stir into it the magnesium flakes until it dissolves.

2.   Combine the rest of the ingredients in a double boiler and stir them until they completely melt and whip them while adding the magnesium mix until you get a creamy mix.

3.   Transfer the lotion into a mason jar and refrigerate it then use it whenever you desire.

4.   This lotion will nourish your skin and make it healthy as well as relieve your body from all the tension and help you sleep well.

Calming Lavender Lotion

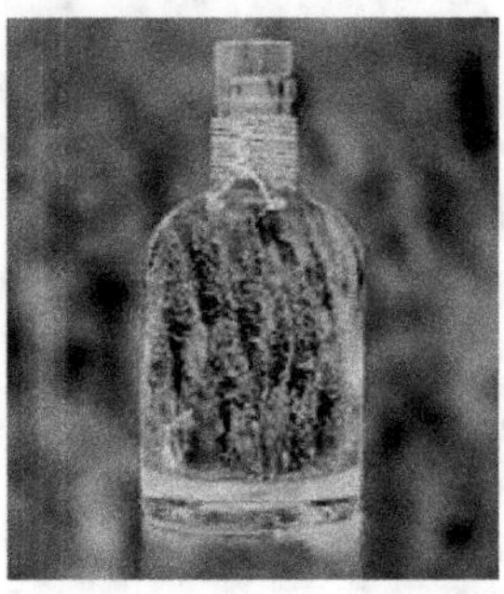

Ingredients:

- ½ cup of organic coconut oil
- 25 drops of lavender essential oil
- 25 drops of Melrose essential oil

Directions:

1.   Melt the coconut oil in a double boiler then stir into it the essential oils and transfer it to a mason jar.

2.   After a long tiring day, this lotion will help you relax and make you feel so good about yourself.

Rosy Shea Lotion

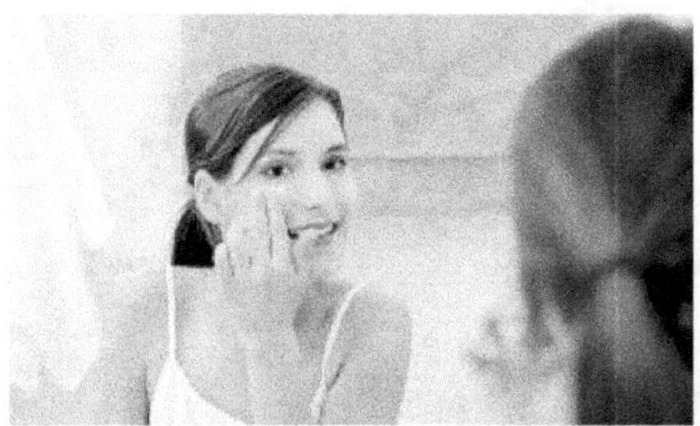

Ingredients:

- ½ cup of shea butter
- 1 tablespoon of almond oil
- 1 tablespoon of jojoba oil
- 10 drops of rosemary essential oil
- 10 drops of lavender essential oil

Directions:

1. Melt the jojoba oil with shea butter and almond oil in a double boiler then refrigerate it for 10 to 15 min.

2. Once the time is up, add in the essential oils and whip the mix with a hand mixer until you get a creamy mix.

3. Transfer your lotion to a mason jar and apply it whenever needed.

4. This lotion will moisturize your skin and prevent it from drying.

Coconut Tea Lotion

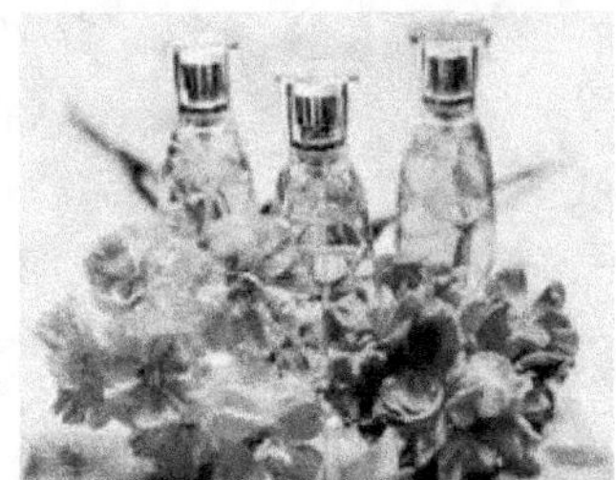

Ingredients:

- ½ cup of shea butter
- 2 tablespoons of avocado oil
- 10 drops of lavender essential oil
- 5 drops of rosemary essential oil
- 3 drops of tea tree essential oil
- 3 drops of carrot seed essential oil

Directions:

1. Melt the avocado oil with shea butter in a double boiler then refrigerate it for 10 to 15 min.

2. Once the time is up, add in the essential oils and whip the mix with a hand mixer until you get a creamy mix.

3. Transfer your lotion to a mason jar and apply it whenever needed.

4. This lotion will moisturize your skin and keep it looking glowing; you can use it on both your body and face.

Non-greasy Cocoa Lotion

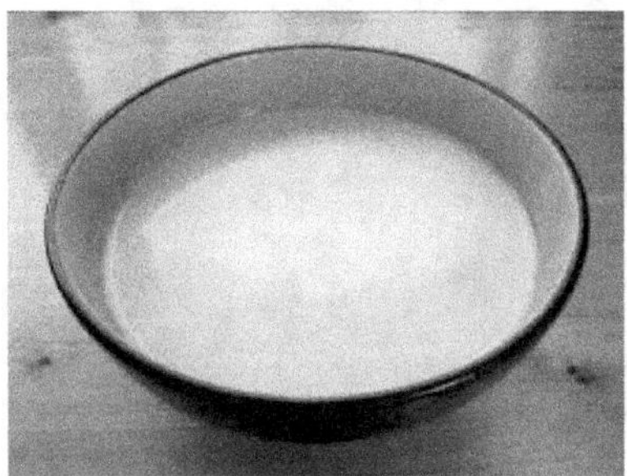

Ingredients:

- ¼ cup of coconut oil
- 1/8 cup of cocoa butter
- 1/8 cup of shea butter
- 1 tablespoon of jojoba oil
- 1 tablespoon of aloe vera juice
- 10 drops of orange essential oil

Directions:

1.   Whisk the essential oil with jojoba oil and aloe vera juice in a small bowl then set it aside.

2.   Combine the rest of the ingredients in a double boiler and melt them completely then stir in the aloe vera mix.

3.   Transfer the lotion into a mason jar and use it whenever you desire.

4.   This lotion will nourish your skin and make it soft.

Creamy Chamomile Lotion

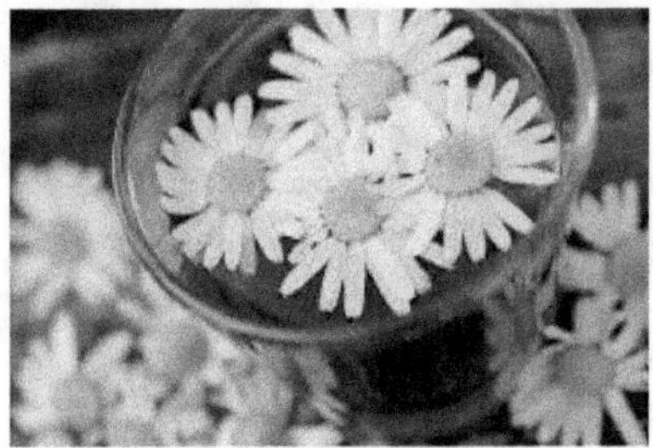

Ingredients:

- 8 ounces of distilled water
- 6 ounces of jojoba oil
- 3 ounces of coconut oil
- 1 ½ ounces of beeswax, grated
- 5 teaspoons of lavender buds
- 5 teaspoons of chamomile flowers

Directions:

1.   Combine the lavender buds with jojoba oil and chamomile flowers in a double boiler then cook them for 2 h on low heat.

2.   Strain the jojoba oil mix through a cheesecloth then combine it with the wax and coconut oil in another double boiler and melt them completely.

3.   Heat the water until it becomes warm to the touch and transfer it into a container then add to it a steady stream of the oils mix while whipping them with an Emerson blender until you get a smooth mix.

4.   Transfer the lotion into a mason jar then use it whenever you want.

5.   This lotion will nourish your skin and soften it as well as calm you and ease all your worries.

Minty Summer Lotion

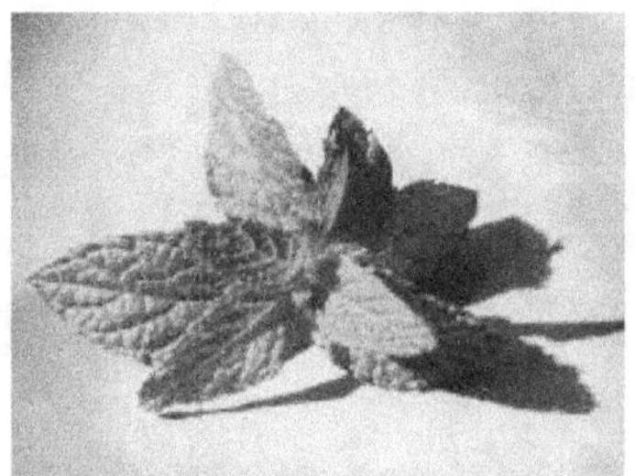

Ingredients:

- ½ cup of aloe vera gel
- ½ cup of coconut oil
- ¼ cup of beeswax, grated
- 1/8 teaspoon of peppermint essential oil

Directions:

1.   Melt the beeswax with coconut oil in a double boiler then whisk in the rest of the ingredients until they become smooth.

2.   Allow the lotion to cool down for 1 h and whisk it again then use it and enjoy.

3.   After a long tiring day in a summer time, this lotion will make you feel cool and keep your skin moisturized.

Eczema Lotion Fighter

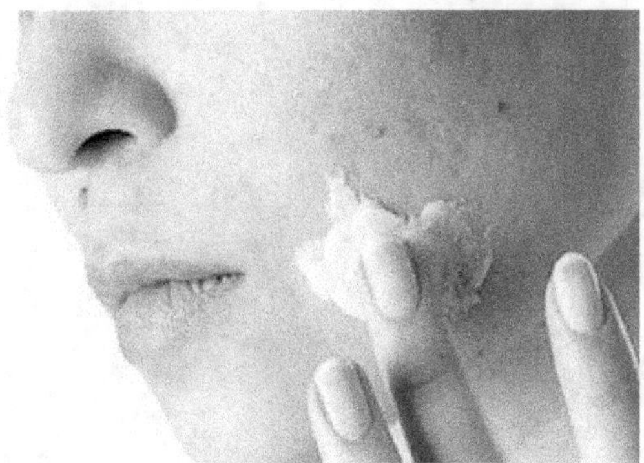

Ingredients:

- ¼ cup of coconut oil
- ¼ cup of shea butter
- 15 drops of lavender essential oil
- 5 drops of tea tree essential oil

Directions:

1. Melt the coconut oil with shea butter in a double boiler then stir into it the essential oils.

2. Transfer the lotion into a mason jar and refrigerate it until it hardens then use it whenever you desire and enjoy.

3. This lotion is high in vitamins so it will contribute to healing your skin from eczema in a fast way.

Creamy Coconut Lotion

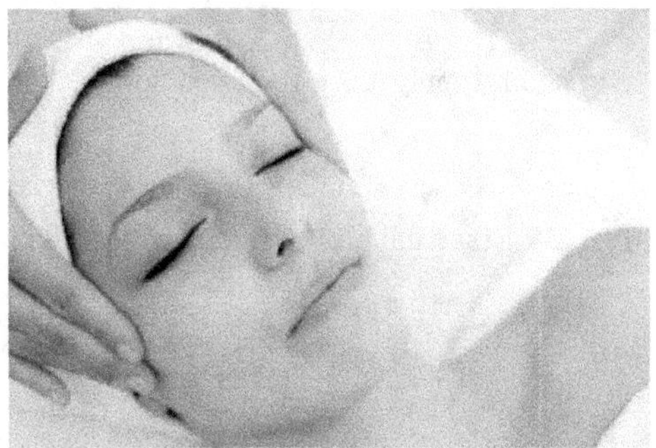

Ingredients:

- ½ cup of beeswax, grated
- ½ cup of fresh aloe vera gel
- ½ cup of distilled water
- ¼ cup of jojoba oil
- ¼ cup of coconut oil
- 1 teaspoon of rosemary extract
- 10 drops of vanilla essential oil
- 5 drops of orange essential oil

Directions:

1. Whisk the water with aloe vera gel and in a bowl and set it aside.

2. Melt the beeswax completely in a double boiler then transfer it with coconut oil, jojoba oil vanilla essential oil, rosemary extract and blend them on the lowest setting.

3.   Add in the aloe vera mix in a steady stream to the oils mix while blending them all the time until you get a smooth and creamy mix.

4.   Transfer the lotion into a mason jar and apply it whenever you desire.

5.   This lotion is not greasy at all, apply whenever you are going it or want to go to the beach, it will keep your skin moisturized and protect it from the sun.

Historical Honey Lotion

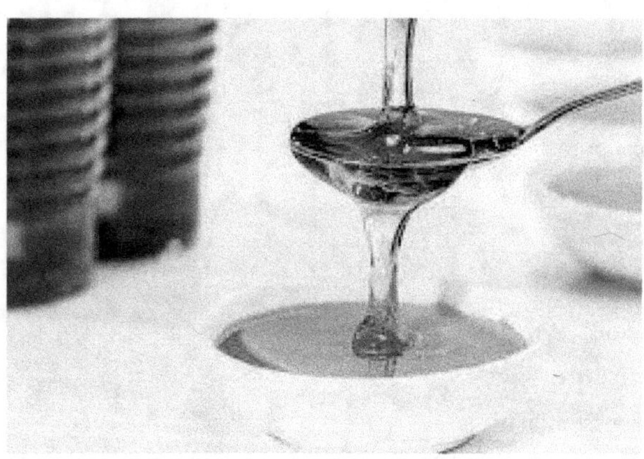

Ingredients:

- 7/8 cups of almond oil
- ½ cup of rose water
- ½ cup tablespoons of beeswax, grated
- 1 tablespoon of raw honey

Directions:

1.   Melt the honey with almond oil and beeswax in a double boiler completely and allow them to cool down for few minutes.

2.   Add the rose water while whisking it all the time then transfer into a mason jar and use it whenever you want.

3.   The lotion will cleanse your face and keep it moisturized.

Wild Rosy Lotion

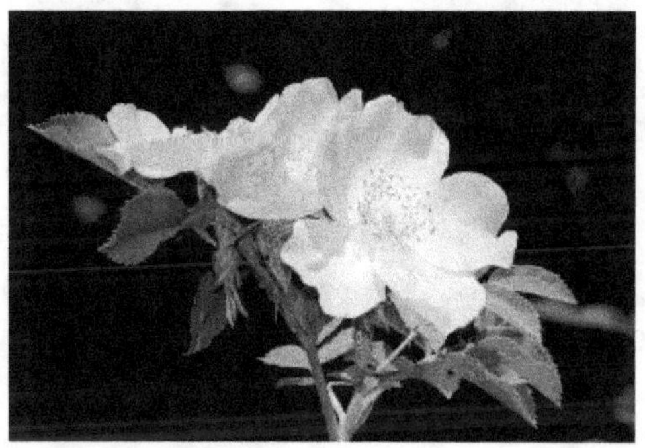

Ingredients:

- 1/3 cup of rosewater
- 1 teaspoon of sunflower oil
- ½ teaspoon of sodium lactate
- ¼ teaspoon of rice bran oil
- ¼ teaspoon of honey

- ¼ teaspoon of liquid Germall plus
- 1/8 teaspoon of cocoa butter
- 20 drops of Vitamin E oil
- 10 drops of geranium essential oil

Directions:

1. Combine the Germall plus, rose water, sodium lactate and honey in a double boiler and melt them completely.

2. Heat the rest ingredients in a double boiler until they become warm to the touch then transfer them with the rose water to a mason jar.

3. Whisk the mix with a coffee whisker until you get a smooth and creamy lotion then refrigerate it and use it whenever you want.

4. This is an amazing hands lotion that will keep your hands soft and make smell good all day.

Chapter 5 – Sunscreen Lotions

Orange Summer Lotion

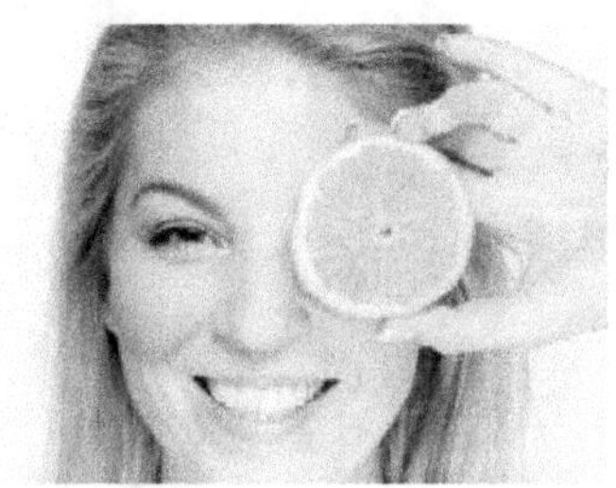

Ingredients:

- ¼ cup of cocoa butter
- 1/8 cup of sweet almond oil
- 1/8 cup of coconut oil
- 25 drops of orange essential oil

Directions:

1. Combine the almond oil with butter and coconut oil in a double boiler and stir them until they completely melt.

2. Remove the oils mix from the heat and stir in the essential oil.

3. Transfer the lotion into a mason jar and allow it to cool down then use it right away or refrigerate it until ready to use.

4. This lotion will moisturize your skin, relieve your stress and make your skin healthier.

Baby Coconut Lotion

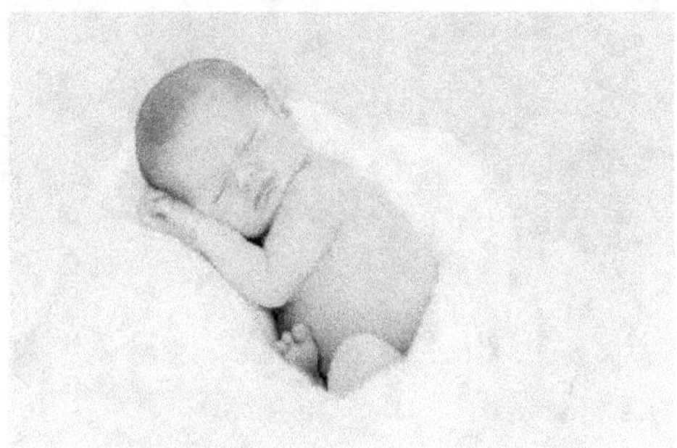

Ingredients:

- 16 ounces of baby lotion
- 8 ounces of vitamin E cream
- 8 ounces of solid coconut oil
- 4 ounces of cocoa butter

Directions:

1.   Combine all the ingredients in a medium bowl and whip them until their soft peaks.

2.   Transfer the mix into a mason jar and seal it then use it right away or refrigerate it until ready to use.

3.   This lotion with make your skin feels amazing.

Aphoristic Lotion

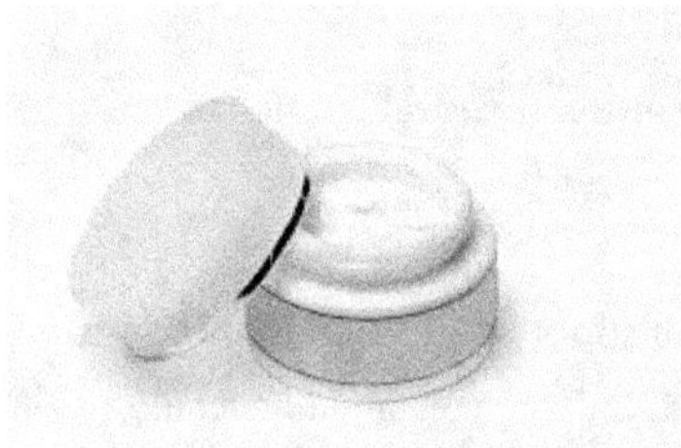

Ingredients:

- ½ cup of grapes seeds oil
- ½ cup of coconut oil
- 1 ounce of beeswax, grated
- ½ ounce of cocoa butter
- ¼ cup of rose hydrosol
- ¼ cup of aloe vera gel
- 1 tablespoon of vitamin E oil
- 1 tablespoon of rosehip seed oil
- 2 teaspoons of Aphrodite aroma oil
- 10 drops of Peru Balsam essential oil

Directions:

1. Combine the grapes seed oil with vitamin E oil, coconut oil, beeswax, cocoa butter with rosehip seed oil in a double boiler then melt them completely.

2. Mix the aloe vera gel with Peru Balsam essential oil in another small bowl then stir them into the oils mix once they cool down and become warm to the touch.

3.   Transfer the mix into a food processor and blend them smooth until the lotion becomes thick like a medium thick pudding.

4.   Stir in the Aphrodite aroma oil into the lotion then transfer it to a mason a jar and refrigerate it or use it right away.

5.   If you want a boost of confidence, or you simply want to impress someone, this lotion will leave your skin soft as a baby's and make you smell heavenly.

Jojoba Nut Lotion

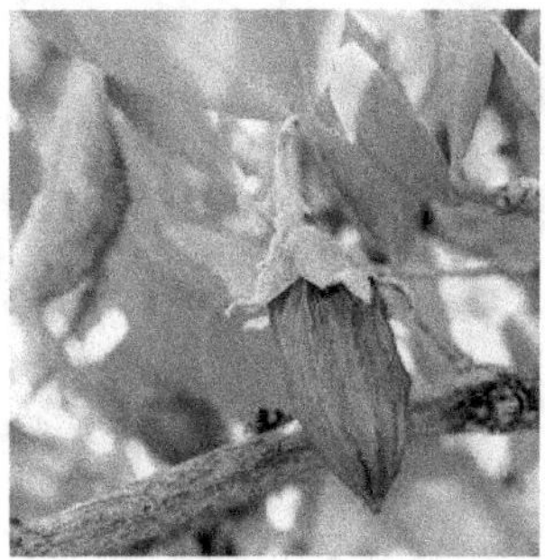

Ingredients:

- ½ cup of jojoba oil
- ½ cup of cocoa butter
- ½ cup of coconut oil

Directions:

1.   Melt the cocoa butter with jojoba oil in a double boiler then stir into them the jojoba oil and remove them from the heat.

2.   Refrigerate the lotion mix for several hours until it starts to firm then whip it with a hand mixer until it becomes creamy.

3.   Transfer the mix into a mason jar and seal it then use it right away or refrigerate it until ready to use.

4.   This lotion will knock off all your store bought lotions and become your favorite because it will moisturize the skin and soften it.

Relaxing Lavender Lotion

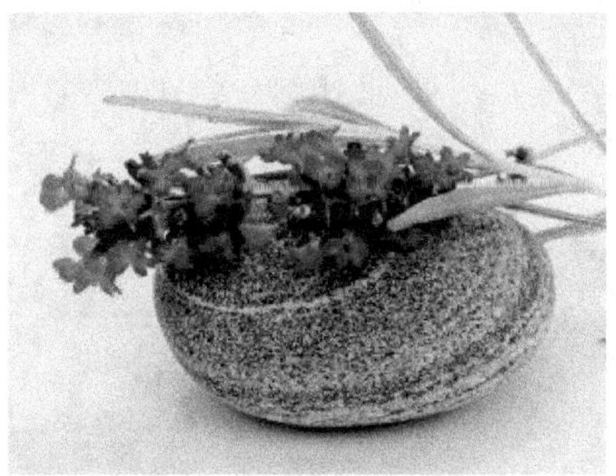

Ingredients:

- 8 ounces of distilled water
- 6 ounces of jojoba oil
- 3 ounces of solid coconut oil
- 1 ½ ounces of beeswax, grated
- 5 drops of chamomile essential oil
- 5 drops of vanilla essential oil

Directions:

1.   Melt the wax with jojoba and coconut oil in a double boiler and stir them until they liquefy.

2.   Heat the water in small saucepan until it becomes warm to the touch then add to it a thin steady stream of oil while whisking all the time with a hand mixer until you get a creamy mix similar to mayonnaise.

3.   Stir in the essential oils and transfer the mix into a mason jar then seal it and use it right away or refrigerate it until ready to use.

4.   After a long tiring day, this lotion removes all the stress from your body as well as helps you relax and sleep better.

Sunny Bee Lotion

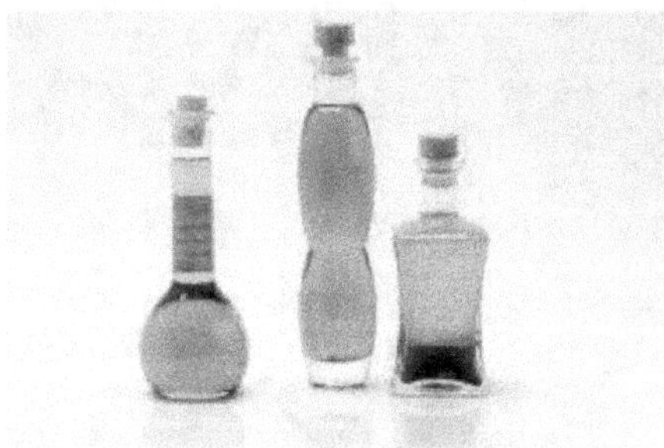

Ingredients:

- ½ cup of sunflower oil
- ¼ cup of boiled water
- 1 tablespoon of beeswax, grated
- 1/8 teaspoon of baking soda

Directions:

1. Pour the water in a small bowl and dissolve in it the baking soda.

2. Combine the wax with oil in a double boiler over low heat and stir it until it completely melts.

3. Heat the soda and water mix until its temperature becomes similar to the oils mix temperature.

4. Pour the soda and water mix into the oils mix in a steady stream while stirring them all the time.

5. Allow the lotion to cool down completely while stirring it every once in a while then transfer it to a mason jar and refrigerate it until you want to use it.

6. This lotion is great for dry skin; it moisturizes it and softens it.

Seductive Vanilla Lotion

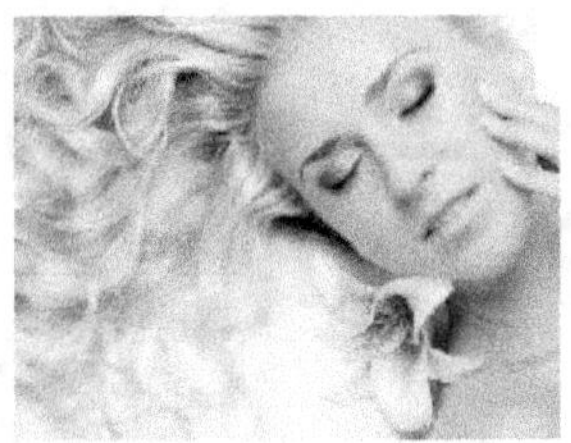

Ingredients:

- ½ cup of olive oil
- ¼ cup of beeswax, grated
- ¼ cup of coconut oil

- 2 tablespoons of cocoa butter
- 1 tablespoon of vitamin E oil
- 2 drops of vanilla extract

Directions:

1. Combine all the ingredients in a mason jar and put on the lid loosely then place it in a double boiler.

2. Stir the mix from time to time with a spoon until it completely melts then use it after taking a bath and enjoy.

3. This lotion will nourish your skin and protect it from eczema; you can use it on your baby as well.

Smooth Clay Lotion

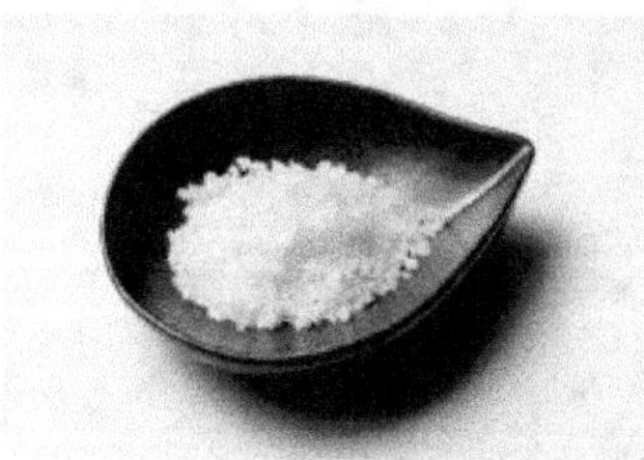

Ingredients:

- 1/8 cup of water
- 1 tablespoon of finely ground sea salt
- 1 tablespoon of baking soda
- 1 tablespoon of bentonite clay
- 1 teaspoon of glycerin

Directions:

1.   Whisk the salt with soda and clay in a small bowl then add in the water followed by the glycerin while whisking all the time until no lumps are found.

2.   Store the lotion in a container and refrigerate it then use it whenever you want and enjoy.

3.   This lotion with smoothen your skin and keeping it from drying.

Sun Blocking lotion

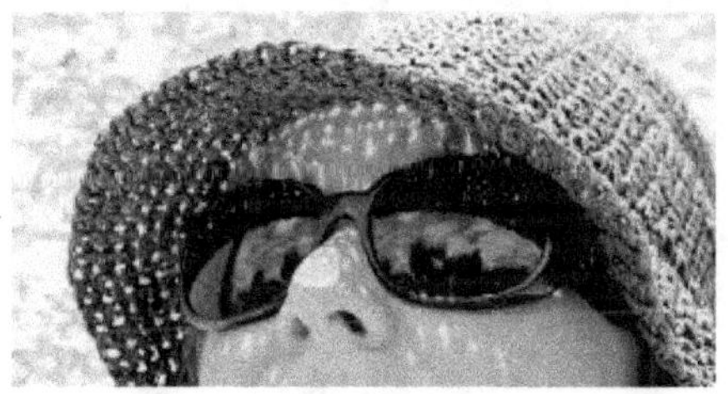

Ingredients:

- 1 ounce of beeswax, grated
- ¼ cup of olive oil
- 2 tablespoons of coconut oil
- 2 teaspoons of shea butter
- 1 teaspoon of vanilla extract

Directions:

1.   Combine the beeswax with coconut oil, butter and olive oil in a double boiler then stir them until they completely melt.

2.   Stir in the vanilla extract into the mix and pour it into a mason jar then use it whenever you want and enjoy.

3.   This lotion will make your skin smooth, protect it from the sun and leave smelling of vanilla.

Natural Sunscreen Lotion

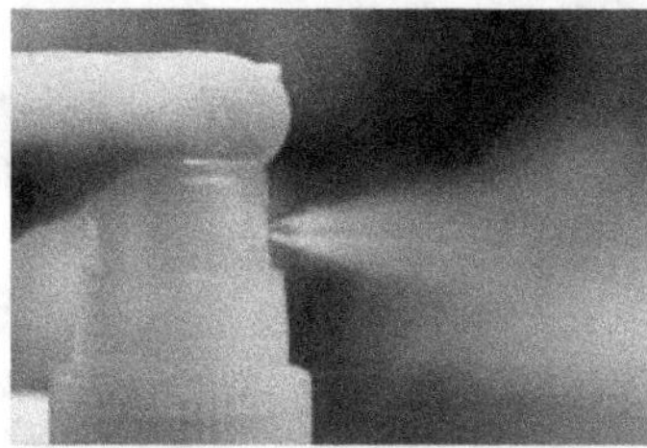

Ingredients:

- 2 ounces of avocado oil
- 2 ounces of beeswax, grated
- 2 ounces of coconut oil
- 1 ounce of shea butter
- 1 ounce of cocoa butter
- 25 drops of lavender essential oil
- 10 drops of carrot seed essential oil
- 10 drops of myrrh essential oil
- 2 drops of sandalwood essential oil

Directions:

1.   Combine all the ingredients except for the essential oils in a double boiler and heat them until they melt completely.

2.   Stir in the vanilla extract into the mix and pour it into a mason jar then use it whenever you want and enjoy.

3.   This lotion will make your skin smooth, nourish it and protect it from the sun.

Aloe Vera Lotion

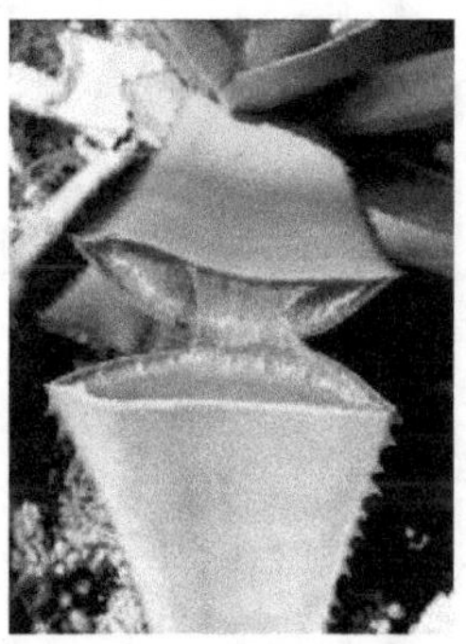

Ingredients:

- 1 cup of pure aloe vera gel
- ½ cup of sweet almond oil
- ½ cup of beeswax, grated
- 1 teaspoon of vitamin E oil
- 15 drops of jasmine essential oil

Directions:

1.	Whisk the essential oil with aloe vera and vitamin E oil in a small bowl and set it aside.

2.	Melt the almond oil with wax in a double boiler then transfer them into a food processor and allow them to cool down for few minutes.

3.	Blend the wax mix on low settings then add in the aloe vera gel gradually while blending them until you are satisfied with the consistency of the lotion.

4.	Transfer the lotion into a mason jar and apply whenever you desire.

5.	This lotion is a great moisturizer for you to use in both summer and winter.

Chapter 6 – Secrets to making natural lotions

If you're like many people who are trending toward more natural health and personal care, learning what's in your lotions and products has become more important than anything else. Here are some secrets to help you make some truly natural lotions and products so you can be sure about what it is you are putting on your skin.

#1: Choosing the Correct Plant

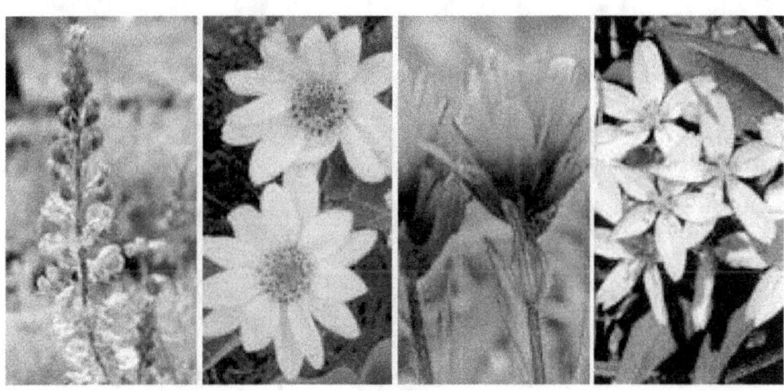

To learn how to make the finest and purest hand-crafted lotions, creams, and skin care products, you first need to know which specific plant ingredients work to balance, repair, and encourage your skin to be its best.

Whether your skin is sensitive, aging, dry, oily, or normal, nature has given us the right plant to correct the problem. Plants all have different properties. Some are astringent or hydrating, others have the ability to absorb moisture or oil, and still others contain properties that mimic human sebum, so choosing the right plant for your skin to include in your homemade lotions is essential.

#2: The Extraction Process

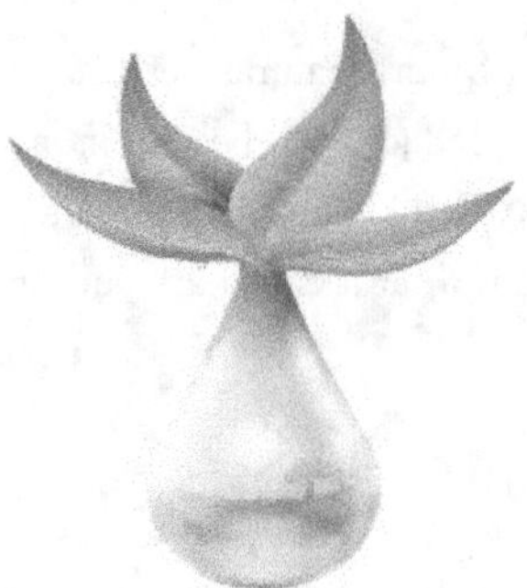

Knowing the properties of plants is the first step to making your own lotions but knowing how to correctly remove those properties from the plant - and which part of the plant to remove them from - is next. Leaves, berries, petals, stems, seeds, and nuts all contribute a specific quality.

Essential oil distillation, infusions, tinctures, decoctions, flower waters, and hydrosols are all used for different reasons in making lotions. They all require differing methods of extraction so the delicate plant properties are not destroyed.

#3: Getting the Desired Texture and Result

Getting oil and water to mix is pure chemistry, but you don't need to be a chemist to keep your lotion ingredients from separating (a process called emulsification). Different consistencies are used for different purposes and the final consistency of your product will be defined as a lotion (hand lotion, body lotion, after shave, cleanser), or a cream (foot cream, eye cream, hand cream, night cream). The result depends on your oil to water ratio and anything less than 20% water will result in an ointment.

There's a lot of information out there about how to take care of your skin and more products than you can ever imagine. Being aware of the characteristics of your skin will go a long way to helping your decide which lotions and products are best for you. Even better, to help you decide which homemade lotion or cream to make for yourself.

Importance of a natural skin lotion

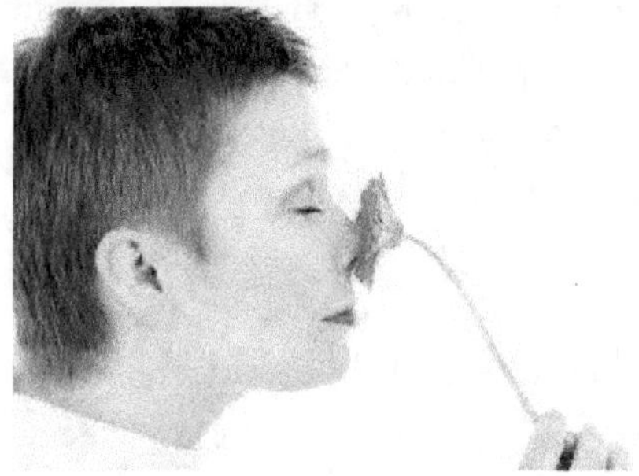

information about an effective and natural skin lotion which can penetrate deep into the skin, nourish it, hydrate it, regenerate it and rejuvenate it. It will also restore the protein balance within the skin. Let us take a look at them one by one.

1. **Nourish and moisturize the skin**- this requirement can be easily met with the natural emollients like Avocado Oil and Maracuja. They have the ability to go deep into the skin and moisturize it inside out. These ingredients have a high nutritional value which is used to nourish the skin and make it healthy from inside.

They also help in regenerating the damaged skin cells, replacing them with the new ones and thus keeping the skin soft, supple and fresh always.

2. **Restore balance among the skin proteins** - this is important to even out the degenerative reactions taking place in the body especially when you are aging. For example - with age, the production of Collagen and Elastin, which are the proteins responsible for keeping the skin smooth and elastic, goes down and hence you develop wrinkles. If you use a lotion containing Cynergy TK(TM), it can restore the level of Collagen and Elastin and make the skin smooth and wrinkle free again.

Similarly, due to the harmful UV rays from the sun, the production of the skin protein called Melanin goes up and as a result it starts depositing in the skin taking the form of age spots. If you use Extrapone Nutgrass Root, it can inhibit the over production of Melanin and thus prevent age spots from occurring.

So essentially, an ideal skin lotion should focus on - one, providing the skin with necessary nutrients to keep it healthy from within; and two, maintaining the balance of skin proteins so that you stay away from common problems like fine lines, wrinkles, age spots, dry skin etc.

If you want to look out for an effective and perfect skin lotion, make sure to check the list of ingredients that it has. It must have some or all of the powerful natural ingredients discussed above.

Conclusion

Standing in the lotion aisle at the market can be overwhelming. Not only are there hundreds of options to choose from, but if you pick up a bottle and try to decipher what it is made of it's like reading a foreign language. Too many lotions and brands use unrecognizable and unpronounceable ingredients.

Most of these ingredients are chemicals, or synthetic materials that were made in a science lab. While they won't give you any harmful diseases, they can cause skin irritation or allergic reactions. Not only that, but they can even dry your skin out more forcing you to constantly reapply and buy bottle after bottle.

If you have sensitive skin or allergies to fragrances or other allergies, trying to decipher the ingredients on the back of the lotion bottle can make the difference between a good experience and a bad one.

The easiest solution is to bypass this entire process. Make your own organic lotion or body butter and rest easy knowing exactly what is in the lotion you are putting on your skin.

Your skin is the largest organ on the body, it is important to take care of it. It is the first line of defense against the environment, and it keeps everything inside our bodies that we want to stay inside our bodies. Your skin is essential, and caring for it properly should be too.

It may seem daunting to try and make your own lotion, but it is as easy as one, two, and three. It is a less stressful solution by far to make your own lotion or body butter, than it is to go through the intense process of buying one.

Making your own lotion, body butter, or hand cream gives you the ability to meet your own specific and unique skin care needs. No one is exactly the same, and therefore no one's skin is the exact same either. Making your own lotion gives you the chance to create a moisturizer for your skin type with the ingredients that will give your skin the health and protection you want it to.

When you make your own lotion, you have the option of mixing as many or as few ingredients as you want. While the recipes above only require two oils and an optional butter, there's no reason you can't add more.

If you wanted the vitamins of Almond oil, the scent and protection of Apricot oil, and the collagen stimulus of Avocado oil, there's no reason you can't have all three. The key is to make sure that you do the math correctly so that your lotion doesn't turn into too much of a liquid and lose that lotion texture.

Some measurements for you:

Three oils:

- ¼ cup each oil for an equal dose of each.
- ½ cup primary oil, 1/8 cup for second and third oils

Four oils:

- ¼ cup primary oil, 1/8 cup for second, third, and fourth oils.

It is not recommended to add more than four oils, not only because the math gets a little trickier after that, but then the mixture might not mix as well and you risk separation.

Have the peace of mind of knowing exactly what you are putting on your body. Take care of your skin; moisturize it, repair it, heal it, and protect it. Lotion can be so much more than just a skin soother, and when you make your own you can make it that way.

Making your own lotion gives you the chance to fight against your biggest skin concerns, whether those are elasticity and collagen concerns, ultraviolet or UV rays concerns, aging and wrinkle concerns, or severe dry skin like eczema. Making your own lotion means you can make the perfect concoction to address all these issues and give yourself beautiful and healthy skin.

Don't settle for store bought lotions which can dry your skin out more or cause allergic reactions or irritation. Make your own and live life in happy, healthy skin.

Thank you again for downloading this book! I do hope you found these recipes as helpful as I did. You can never go wrong with organic and natural products, and the results will always be surprisingly incredible!!